WEIGHT CUTTING FOR FIGHTING

WEIGHT CUTTING FOR FIGHTING

BEN ZEE

For information about this title, contact the publisher:

Coach Ben Zee
coachbz.com
benzhuang1@gmail.com

ISBNs:
979-8-9874863-0-6 (hardcover)
979-8-9874863-1-3 (softcover)
979-8-9874863-2-0 (eBook)

Printed in the United States of America

Cover and Interior design: 1106 Design

CONTENTS

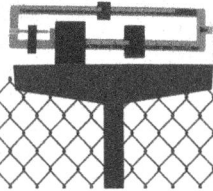

0. DISCLAIMER

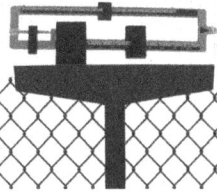

Weight cutting can be dangerous. Losing drastic amounts of weight can and has resulted in permanent bodily harm and death. Individuals under the age of 18 should not cut weight. Always consult your physician, and use safe weight-management practices under the supervision of a professional. None of this is medical advice, and the author is not liable for outcomes. If anything goes wrong, immediately call for emergency services.

Be responsible, and keep in mind that this was written for combat-sports athletes. The weight-cutting protocols for physique competitions are vastly different. The goal here is not to look better in the mirror. It is to make the agreed-upon weight as safely as possible, and then perform optimally. Weight cutting is not always a fun experience, and you must mentally prepare yourself for that reality. But for now, it is a part of the game.

1. INTRODUCTION

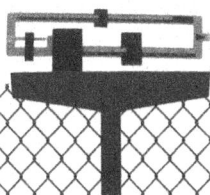

M aking weight for competition is about losing weight in the short-term, or "acute weight loss." By using strategies for acute weight loss during the final week before weigh-in, you are able to potentially gain a competitive advantage. Acute weight loss includes losing fluids, removing gut contents, and glycogen depletion. These strategies allow you to rapidly decrease your body weight, weigh in, and then replace what you lost before competition. Acute weight loss is different from long-term or chronic weight loss, where the goal is to lose fat and/or muscle. Chronic weight loss is a much slower process and is covered briefly in the preparation phase.

When it comes to weight-class sports, you must understand how to effectively make weight. Done wrong, weight cutting can lead to disaster. But done correctly, weight cutting can give an athlete a significant competitive advantage. This advantage is greater in combat sports, such as wrestling, where the goal is to impose your body weight on your opponent. This advantage is lesser in striking arts, such as boxing, which has minimal grappling and more space to move. In mixed martial arts, the heavier athlete tends to be more powerful and has an advantage in the clinch, cage work, and grappling. But there can also be benefits for the lighter athlete, such as speed and conditioning.

2. AUTHOR

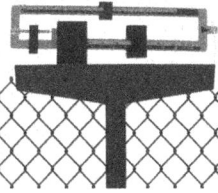

Coach Ben is a Performance Coach and Jiu-Jitsu Instructor based in Los Angeles, California. He works with athletes in the UFC, PFL, Bellator, ONE, NHL, and professional boxing.

3. OVERVIEW

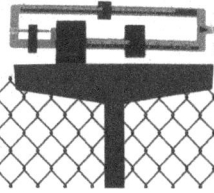

The amount of weight you can safely cut depends on your body weight and the amount of time you have to recover post-weigh-in. Less time to recover means that less weight can be cut.

The following are the most common scenarios:

1. ≥ 24 HOUR WEIGH-IN
Typically used in Professional MMA
24 hours or more to recover after weigh-in

2. = 6 TO 12 HOUR WEIGH-IN
Typically used in Judo and Amateur MMA
Between 6 and 12 hours to recover after weigh-in

3. ≤ 2 HOUR WEIGH-IN
Typically used in Jiu-Jitsu and Grappling
2 hours or less to recover after weigh-in

Once the proper weight class is determined, use the following system:

Phase 1: Preparation
Phase 2: Weight Cut
Phase 3: Post-Weigh-In

PHASE 1: PREPARATION

Ideally 8 to 12+ weeks out.

During the preparation phase, you want to prioritize **losing body fat, gaining muscle mass, and heat acclimation**. Losing body fat is a process that must be done over time. If you try to aggressively lose body fat, your performance will suffer, and you risk losing lean muscle mass. Gaining muscle mass can benefit performance, and having more muscle allows you to cut more water weight via dehydration. The body stores plenty of water in muscle tissue, while almost none is stored in fat cells. Heat acclimation trains your body to sweat and benefits performance. All of these things require time, and, in an ideal situation, you have a full 8 to 12+ weeks for the preparation phase. For short-notice competitions with less than two weeks before weigh-in day, skip Phase 1 and go directly to Phase 2.

PHASE 2: WEIGHT CUT

Ideally 5 to 7+ days out.

Fiber Elimination
Glycogen Depletion
Water Loading
Sodium Reduction
Active/Passive Dehydration

The second phase begins roughly a week before weigh-in. You generally begin the weight-cut phase 5 to 7 days out from weigh-in day. The more weight an athlete has to lose, the more additional mechanisms must be used. Whether some or all of the mechanics are used depends on the individual. The main focus of the weight cut is to manipulate water and gut contents within the body. When this is done effectively, it causes a rapid decrease in body weight.

You want to temporarily reduce water stored in the body and gut contents stored in the intestines. Especially in the final days prior to weigh-in, you want to **consume food that is low in fiber**. Excessive fiber intake will cause the body to retain water, while eliminating fiber does the opposite and causes the body to lose water. As you get closer to weigh-in day, you also want to begin consuming foods that are light in actual weight.

Utilizing a low-carbohydrate diet will cause **glycogen depletion** to occur in the body. The body responds to this by losing water rapidly. When on a low-carb diet, consume a larger percentage of protein, and avoid consuming high amounts of dietary fat. Consuming a high-fat diet can be detrimental to performance.

On the days leading up to the weigh-in, a **water-loading protocol** is used to encourage body-water loss and help with satiety. In addition, **decreasing sodium intake** can further reduce water stored in the body. The final portion of the weight-cut phase involves **dehydration via the use of active and/or passive sweating methods**. This is the final step prior to stepping on the official scale to weigh in.

PHASE 3: POST-WEIGH-IN

0 to 36 hours out.

Replenish fluids and electrolytes
Replenish carbohydrates
Consume low-fat and low-fiber foods
Continue drinking fluids and monitor hydration status

After successfully weighing in, **replenish fluids and electrolytes**. Then **replenish carbohydrates** by **consuming low-fat and low-fiber foods**. Avoid consuming anything that can be detrimental to performance, and avoid trying new and unfamiliar things. Throughout Phase 3, **continue drinking fluids and monitor hydration status**.

4. WEIGHT CLASS

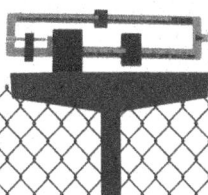

Most combat sports involve weight classes. The following charts can be used as a guide to determine where you have to be in order to compete in a certain weight class. The charts are based off of the 3 common scenarios covered in the beginning of the previous chapter.

≥ 24 HOUR WEIGH-IN

For competitions that allow 24 hours or more to recover after weigh-in, aim to get to within **6%** to **8%** more than but no more than **10%** more than the contracted weight 5 days before weigh-in.

EXAMPLE: An athlete competing in the 171-pound weight class will ideally weigh between 181.3 and 184.7, and no more than 188.1 pounds on *Sunday* morning if their weigh-in is the following *Friday* morning. Athletes competing in the UFC generally compete 30–36 hours after weighing in and would fall into this category.

UFC Title Fights in Pounds

115 lbs.—121.9 to 124.2; no more than **126.5**
125 lbs.—132.5 to 135.0; no more than **137.5**
135 lbs.—143.1 to 145.8; no more than **148.5**
145 lbs.—153.7 to 156.6; no more than **159.5**
155 lbs.—164.3 to 167.4; no more than **170.5**
170 lbs.—180.2 to 183.6; no more than **187.0**
185 lbs.—196.1 to 199.8; no more than **203.5**
205 lbs.—217.3 to 221.4; no more than **225.5**
265 lbs.—280.9 to 286.2; no more than **291.5**

UFC Title Fights in Kilograms

52.2 kg—55.3 to 56.4; no more than **57.4**
56.7 kg—60.1 to 61.2; no more than **62.4**
61.2 kg—64.9 to 66.1; no more than **67.3**
65.8 kg—69.7 to 71.1; no more than **72.4**
70.3 kg—74.5 to 75.9; no more than **77.3**
77.1 kg—81.7 to 83.3; no more than **84.8**
83.9 kg—88.9 to 90.6; no more than **92.3**
93.0 kg—98.6 to 100.4; no more than **102.3**
120.2 kg—127.4 to 129.8; no more than **132.2**

UFC Non-Title Fights in Pounds

116 lbs.—123.0 to 125.3; no more than **127.6**
126 lbs.—133.6 to 136.1; no more than **138.6**
136 lbs.—144.2 to 146.9; no more than **149.6**
146 lbs.—154.8 to 157.7; no more than **160.6**
156 lbs.—165.4 to 168.5; no more than **171.6**

171 lbs.—181.3 to 184.7; no more than **188.1**
186 lbs.—197.2 to 200.9; no more than **204.6**
206 lbs.—218.4 to 222.5; no more than **226.6**
266 lbs.—282.0 to 287.3; no more than **292.6**

UFC Non-Title Fights in Kilograms

52.6 kg—55.8 to 56.8; no more than **57.9**
57.2 kg—60.6 to 61.8; no more than **62.9**
61.7 kg—65.4 to 66.6; no more than **67.9**
66.2 kg—70.2 to 71.5; no more than **72.8**
70.8 kg—75.0 to 76.5; no more than **77.9**
77.6 kg—82.3 to 83.8; no more than **85.4**
84.4 kg—89.5 to 91.2; no more than **92.8**
93.4 kg—99.0 to 100.9; no more than **102.7**
120.6 kg—127.8 to 130.2; no more than **132.7**

≥ 6 TO 12 HOUR WEIGH-IN

For competitions that allow 6 to 12 hours to recover after weigh-in, aim to get to within **2%** to **4%** more than but no more than **5%** more than the contracted weight 5 days before weigh-in.

EXAMPLE: An athlete competing in the 171-pound weight class will ideally weigh between 174.4 and 177.8 but no more than 179.6 pounds on *Monday* morning if their weigh-in is the following *Saturday* morning. Athletes competing in certain amateur MMA or Judo events compete 6 to 12 hours after weighing in and would fall into this category. This can be applied to most events where you have morning weigh-in and afternoon or evening competition.

Amateur MMA Fights in Pounds
116 lbs.—118.3 to 120.6; no more than **121.8**
126 lbs.—128.5 to 131.0; no more than **132.3**
136 lbs.—138.7 to 141.4; no more than **142.8**
146 lbs.—148.9 to 151.8; no more than **153.3**
156 lbs.—159.1 to 162.2; no more than **163.8**
171 lbs.—174.4 to 177.8; no more than **179.6**
186 lbs.—189.7 to 193.4; no more than **195.3**
206 lbs.—210.1 to 214.2; no more than **216.3**
266 lbs.—271.3 to 276.6; no more than **279.3**

Amateur MMA Fights in Kilograms
52.6 kg—53.7 to 54.7; no more than **55.2**
57.2 kg—58.3 to 59.5; no more than **60.1**
61.7 kg—62.9 to 64.2; no more than **64.8**
66.2 kg—67.5 to 68.8; no more than **69.5**
70.8 kg—72.2 to 73.6; no more than **74.3**
77.6 kg—79.2 to 80.7; no more than **81.5**
84.4 kg—86.1 to 87.8; no more than **88.6**
93.4 kg—95.3 to 97.1; no more than **98.1**
120.6 kg—123.0 to 125.4; no more than **126.6**

≤ 2 HOUR WEIGH-IN
For competitions that allow 2 or fewer hours to recover after weigh-in, aim to get to within **0%** to **2%** more than but no

more than **3%** more than the contracted weight 5 days before weigh-in. For competitions with multiple day weigh-ins, you also want to be within this range.

EXAMPLE: An athlete competing in the 168-pound weight class will ideally weigh between 168.0 and 171.4 but no more than 173.0 pounds on *Monday* morning if their weigh-in is the following *Saturday* morning. Athletes competing in grappling competitions generally compete 0–2 hours after weighing-in and would fall into this category. This can be applied to most events where you weigh-in and compete almost immediately.

IBJJF Jiu-Jitsu (Gi) Competition in Pounds

MALE
127.0 lbs.—127.0 to 129.5; no more than **130.8**
141.6 lbs.—141.6 to 144.4; no more than **145.8**
154.6 lbs.—154.6 to 157.7; no more than **159.2**
168.0 lbs.—168.0 to 171.4; no more than **173.0**
181.6 lbs.—181.6 to 185.2; no more than **187.0**
195.0 lbs.—195.0 to 198.9; no more than **200.9**
208.0 lbs.—208.0 to 212.2; no more than **214.2**
222.0 lbs.—222.0 to 226.4; no more than **228.7**

FEMALE
107.0 lbs.—107.0 to 109.1; no more than **110.2**
118.0 lbs.—118.0 to 120.4; no more than **121.5**

129.0 lbs.—129.0 to 131.6; no more than **132.9**
141.6 lbs.—141.6 to 144.4; no more than **145.8**
152.6 lbs.—152.6 to 155.7; no more than **157.2**
163.6 lbs.—163.6 to 166.9; no more than **168.5**
175.0 lbs.—175.0 to 178.5; no more than **180.3**

IBJJF Jiu-Jitsu (Gi) Competition in Kilograms

MALE
57.5 kg—57.5 to 58.7; no more than **59.2**
64.0 kg—64.0 to 65.3; no more than **65.9**
70.0 kg—70.0 to 71.4; no more than **72.1**
76.0 kg—76.0 to 77.5; no more than **78.3**
82.3 kg—82.3 to 83.9; no more than **84.8**
88.3 kg—88.3 to 90.1; no more than **90.9**
94.3 kg—94.3 to 96.2; no more than **97.1**
100.5 kg—100.5 to 102.5; no more than **103.5**

FEMALE
48.5 kg—48.5 to 49.5; no more than **50.0**
53.5 kg—53.5 to 54.6; no more than **55.1**
58.5 kg—58.5 to 59.7; no more than **60.3**
64.0 kg—64.0 to 65.3; no more than **65.9**
69.0 kg—69.0 to 70.4; no more than **71.1**
74.0 kg—74.0 to 75.5; no more than **76.2**
79.3 kg—79.3 to 80.9; no more than **81.7**

IBJJF Jiu-Jitsu (NoGi) Competition in Pounds

MALE
122.6 lbs.—122.6 to 125.1; no more than **126.3**
136.0 lbs.—136.0 to 138.7; no more than **140.1**
149.0 lbs.—149.0 to 152.0; no more than **153.5**
162.6 lbs.—162.6 to 165.9; no more than **167.5**
175.6 lbs.—175.6 to 179.1; no more than **180.9**
188.6 lbs.—188.6 to 192.3; no more than **194.3**
202.0 lbs.—202.0 to 206.0; no more than **208.1**
215.0 lbs.—215.0 to 219.3; no more than **221.5**

FEMALE
103.0 lbs.—103.0 to 105.1; no more than **106.1**
114.0 lbs.—114.0 to 116.3; no more than **117.4**
125.0 lbs.—125.0 to 127.5; no more than **128.8**
136.0 lbs.—136.0 to 138.7; no more than **140.1**
147.0 lbs.—147.0 to 149.9; no more than **151.4**
158.0 lbs.—158.0 to 161.2; no more than **162.7**
169.0 lbs.—169.0 to 172.4; no more than **174.1**

IBJJF Jiu-Jitsu (NoGi) Competition in Kilograms

MALE
55.6 kg—55.6 to 56.7; no more than **57.3**
61.7 kg—61.7 to 62.9; no more than **63.6**
67.5 kg—67.5 to 68.9; no more than **69.5**
73.5 kg—73.5 to 75.0; no more than **75.7**

79.6 kg—79.6 to 81.2; no more than **82.0**
85.5 kg—85.5 to 87.2; no more than **88.1**
91.6 kg—91.6 to 93.4; no more than **94.3**
97.5 kg—97.5 to 99.5; no more than **100.4**

FEMALE
46.7 kg—46.7 to 47.6; no more than **48.1**
51.7 kg—51.7 to 52.7; no more than **53.3**
56.7 kg—56.7 to 57.8; no more than **58.4**
61.6 kg—61.6 to 62.8; no more than **63.4**
66.7 kg—66.7 to 68.0; no more than **68.7**
71.6 kg—71.6 to 73.0; no more than **73.7**
76.6 kg—76.6 to 78.1; no more than **78.9**

ADCC World Championship in Pounds

MALE
-145.2 lbs.—145.2 to 148.1; no more than **149.6**
-169.5 lbs.—169.5 to 172.9; no more than **174.6**
-193.7 lbs.—193.7 to 197.6; no more than **199.5**
-218.0 lbs.—218.0 to 222.4; no more than **224.5**
+218.0 lbs.—**no weight limit**

FEMALE
-121.2 lbs.—121.2 to 123.6; no more than **124.8**
-143.3 lbs.—143.3 to 146.2; no more than **147.6**
+143.3 lbs.—**no weight limit**

ADCC World Championship in Kilograms

MALE

-66 kg—66.0 to 67.4; no more than **68.0**
-77 kg—77.0 to 78.6; no more than **79.4**
-88 kg—88.0 to 89.8; no more than **90.7**
-99 kg—99.0 to 101.0; no more than **102.0**
+99 kg—no weight limit

FEMALE

-55 kg—55.0 to 56.1; no more than **56.7**
-65 kg—65.0 to 66.3; no more than **67.0**
+65 kg—no weight limit

MOVING TO A LOWER WEIGHT CLASS

Moving down to a lower weight class is about how much body fat you can potentially lose. It is preferable to lose primarily fat as opposed to muscle when moving down weight classes. Consider moving to a lower weight class if you are not cutting much weight or if you are undersized for your weight class.

For male combat-sports athletes, do not go lower than 6% body fat. For female combat-sports athletes, do not go lower than 12% body fat. If, after checking your body-fat percentage, you still have a good amount of body fat that you could lose before reaching that threshold, then you could potentially move to a lower weight class.

MOVING TO A HIGHER WEIGHT CLASS

Moving up to a higher weight class is about how much muscle you can potentially gain. It is preferable to gain primarily muscle as opposed to fat when moving up weight classes. Consider moving to a higher weight class if you are very lean already and cutting a large amount of weight. If you already struggle to make weight and you are big for the weight class, then you could potentially move to a higher weight class.

You can determine how much potential you have to gain muscle by going online and using a maximum muscular body-weight calculator.

5. PHASE 1: PREPARATION

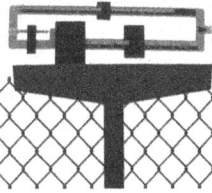

IDEALLY 8 TO 12+ WEEKS

During the preparation phase, the two priorities are: **losing body fat**, **gaining lean muscle mass**, and **heat acclimation**. Losing body fat and gaining lean muscle mass is generally going to improve performance, and more muscle mass allows more water to be removed via dehydration. Muscle contains roughly 75% water, while fat contains only about 10%. At a minimum, maintain lean muscle mass, and avoid excessive body-fat gain between competitions. Preparation for the weight cut also involves heat acclimation, which is a process that gets your body accustomed to tolerating higher temperatures.

Use the guidelines below to determine if you are within the proper weight at the beginning of camp. If you are not within the guidelines, more time is needed, or you must move to a heavier division.

At the Start of an 8-week camp, be within:
15% of weigh-in weight for ≥ 24 hour weigh-in
8% of weigh-in weight for = 6 to 12 hour weigh-in
6% of weigh-in weight for ≤ 2 hour weigh-in

1. LOSING BODY FAT/GAINING LEAN MUSCLE MASS

In an ideal situation, you have at least 8 to 12 weeks to condition your body for competition. Leaner athletes tend to sweat more, and improving body composition can also improve performance. Even for a short-notice competition, losing body fat can be effective, as long as there is a minimum of 2 weeks' notice. When there is less than 2 weeks' notice, focus on the methods used in Phases 2 and 3.

Assuming There Is Still Fat to Lose

During the preparation phase, the idea is to decrease body fat percentage while increasing lean muscle mass. For athletes who begin camp with relatively low body-fat percentage, focus on maintaining rather than gaining additional muscle mass.

Body Fat Guidelines
Men: 6% to 15% body fat
Women: 15% to 25% body fat

Focus on losing .5% to 1% of total body weight per week. A .5% loss is considered "moderate," and a 1% loss is considered "aggressive." To accomplish this with training, increase energy expenditure and/or training duration. To accomplish this with diet, reduce total daily calories by 15% ("moderate") to 25% ("aggressive"). **Experiment by using a combination of both to find what is optimal for you.**

2. HEAT ACCLIMATION

Heat acclimation involves acclimating the body to heat stress by being in a heated environment. Sweating will be more rapid and occur earlier when the body is acclimated to heat stress. Glycogen utilization is also improved, as the body begins to use fatty acids for energy instead of glycogen during times of heat stress. This mechanism allows your body to retain more electrolytes through sweat loss. This improves energy utilization and can make the weight cut less challenging, both physically and mentally. Heat acclimation also creates heat-shock proteins and increases blood-plasma volume. This can lead to an increase in cardiac output and an overall increase in performance.

GUIDELINES

Heat acclimation occurs when you raise your core temperature past 38.5 degrees. This can be achieved by passively sitting in a sauna or hot bath. Start off with no more than 10–20 minutes. These sessions should be relaxing, and there should not be any intense discomfort. Slowly increase the duration of your heat-acclimation sessions as your heat tolerance increases. Build up to 30+ minute sessions, experiment with what you are comfortable with, and do not exceed 1 hour.

Be sure to drink fluids and stay hydrated during heat-acclimation sessions. The purpose is not to dehydrate the body but rather to get the body accustomed to heat stress on a consistent basis. There is no reason to leave the body in a dehydrated state until the end stages of Phase 2.

Begin heat acclimation at least 2 to 3 weeks out from weigh-in.

6. PHASE 2: WEIGHT CUT

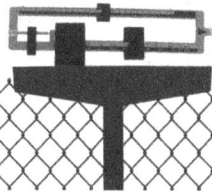

IDEALLY, 5 TO 10 DAYS

The actual "weight cut," not including preparation, typically begins around 5 days out from weigh-in day. For a Friday weigh-in, Phase 2 begins on the previous Sunday. This can be extended 6 to 10 days out from weigh-in day, depending on the amount of weight you must lose. Additional time also allows for you to begin glycogen depletion earlier if needed.

METHODS

1. Athlete's Preferences
2. Gut-Content Elimination
3. Glycogen Depletion
4. Water Loading
5. Sodium Restriction
6. Dehydration

Each method can each be used independently of the others. For example, if an athlete is very close to their weigh-in weight with 5 days left to go, using only gut-content elimination and dehydration may be enough.

Using fewer methods exposes the body to fewer stressors and potential complications. Using more methods allows the body to lose more weight and can make things easier overall.

For example, most professional MMA athletes tend to use all of the methods, due to the amount of time they have to recover. While a jiu-jitsu athlete who competes immediately after weigh-in may use only gut-content elimination, water loading, and dehydration.

Individual response can vary greatly. At the end of the day, it is most effective for each athlete to experiment and develop a personalized system.

1. ATHLETE'S PREFERENCES

Individual preferences of the athlete must be considered, as long as they are within reason. Athletes' preferences include things such as preferred foods, specific brands, sweating methods, or other rituals. For example, some athletes prefer using a sauna, whereas others prefer the using a hot bath. Some athletes also don't enjoy eating certain foods. As always, it is best to avoid adding new methods that haven't been previously tested.

2. GUT-CONTENT ELIMINATION

You can store several pounds of weight in gut contents, depending on your size. Those who regularly consume a high-fiber diet, consisting of lots of vegetables and whole grains will lose more weight from eliminating fiber, compared to those who do not. Fiber is the undigestible parts of fruits, vegetables, and grains. It is technically a carbohydrate but can be digested only by the bacteria produced in your colon. 20g to 40g of fiber per day is recommended for *general* health—when not attempting to make weight. A low-fiber diet decreases stool bulk and limits the amount of undigested material in the large intestine. Most importantly, fiber does not need to be replaced prior to competition and has no effects on performance. Eliminating fiber is essentially free weight loss.

Medically, a low-fiber diet is considered to be between 10g and 15g of fiber per day. In order to eliminate gut contents, use a very-low-fiber diet, consisting of **no more than 10g of fiber per day**. It is difficult to completely eliminate fiber from your diet, but any fiber consumed should be in the form of soluble as opposed to insoluble fiber. Fiber retains water and also slows down the passing of ingested food. Staying on a low-fiber diet for at least 3 days will maximize weight lost due to gut-content elimination; 3 to 4 days is preferred, with a minimum of 2 days needed for any noticeable results. In addition to consuming foods low in fiber, consume foods that are low in weight/volume as you get closer to weigh-in day.

After weigh-in, do not consume too much fiber too rapidly. Excessive fiber intake can impede the absorption of other, more-essential nutrients. Consuming too much fiber after a period of restriction can also cause diarrhea and gastrointestinal distress.

3. GLYCOGEN DEPLETION

The purpose of a low-carb diet for making weight is to deplete glycogen stores in the body. Doing so can cause a significant loss of body water and body weight within a short period of time. Typically, this is achieved by **consuming no more than 50g of carbohydrates per day, for 3 to 4 days**.

Carbohydrates are broken down from the foods you eat and converted into glucose. Glucose is the main source of fuel for cells in the body. When glucose isn't used immediately, it is stored in the liver and muscles as glycogen, to act as a stored form of carbohydrates. When the body needs energy and glucose isn't readily available, glycogen is broken down to be used as fuel. Depending on your size and how well-trained you are, the muscles store 400–800 grams of glycogen, and the liver stores 80–120 grams of glycogen.

Glycogen, however, causes the body to retain water, and 1g of glycogen equates to about 3g of water in the body. Consuming fewer than 50g of carbohydrates per day will cause the body to rapidly lose water weight. When doing this, most of your carbohydrate intake will go toward bodily functions as opposed to fully replenishing glycogen stores.

So most of the carbohydrates should be consumed prior to training or physical activity. When done properly, glycogen depletion is an effective way to lose 2–3% of your body weight in a short period of time.

4. WATER LOADING

Another method for acute weight loss is water loading. Water loading consists of drinking a larger volume of water per day than you are accustomed to. **For most people, this is going to be around 2 gallons or 7.6 liters.** Sustain this for several days, and follow up with a day of fluid restriction, where you eliminate water until weigh-in. Drinking a large amount of water for several days up-regulates body processes responsible for urine production. There is no consensus on the mechanisms of water loading. It's a complicated science involving ADH, aldosterone, vasopressin, aquaporin channels, etc. It *is* effective, however, and has been safely used by athletes to make weight. Water loading also assists with gut-content elimination.

WARNING: If you have any irregular symptoms or do not feel well, stop water loading immediately, and consult your physician. Do not drink more than 32 ounces of water in one sitting; spread out your water intake throughout the day. Remember that body weight will initially increase when you begin water loading. This is normal. Do not let that alarm you, and remember that every gallon of water weighs 8.35 pounds. Every liter of water weighs 2.2 pounds. This is temporary fluid within the body and does not count toward overall body mass.

WATER-LOADING PROTOCOL

Use your current body weight in kilograms (kg) when calculating water intake for water loading.

Kilograms (kg) = Pounds Divided by 2.205

Day 1—Body weight in kg x .10 = water intake in liters
Day 2—Body weight in kg x .10 = water intake in liters
Day 3—Body weight in kg x .10 = water intake in liters
Day 4—Body weight in kg x .10 = water intake in liters
Day 5—Body weight in kg x .01 = water intake in liters
Day 6—No water until weighed in

Example for a 200-lb. or a 90.7-kg athlete:

Day 1—90.7 multiplied by .10 = 9.1 liters or 2.4 gallons
Day 2—90.7 multiplied by .10 = 9.1 liters or 2.4 gallons
Day 3—90.7 multiplied by .10 = 9.1 liters or 2.4 gallons
Day 4—90.7 multiplied by .10 = 9.1 liters or 2.4 gallons
Day 5—90.7 multiplied by .01 = .91 liters or 31 fluid ounces
Day 6—No water until weighed in

Water-Loading Weight Chart (Gallons/Fluid Ounces)

120 lbs./54.4 kg—Days 1 to 4: 1.44 gal | Day 5: 18.4 fl. oz.
130 lbs./59.0 kg—Days 1 to 4: 1.56 gal | Day 5: 20.0 fl. oz.
140 lbs./63.5 kg—Days 1 to 4: 1.68 gal | Day 5: 21.5 fl. oz.

150 lbs./68.0 kg—Days 1 to 4: 1.80 gal | Day 5: 23.0 fl. oz.

160 lbs./72.6 kg—Days 1 to 4: 1.92 gal | Day 5: 25.5 fl. oz.

170 lbs./77.1 kg—Days 1 to 4: 2.04 gal | Day 5: 26.1 fl. oz.

180 lbs./81.6 kg—Days 1 to 4: 2.16 gal | Day 5: 27.6 fl. oz.

190 lbs./86.2 kg—Days 1 to 4: 2.28 gal | Day 5: 29.1 fl. oz.

200 lbs./90.7 kg—Days 1 to 4: 2.40 gal | Day 5: 31.0 fl. oz.

210 lbs./95.2 kg—Days 1 to 4: 2.51 gal | Day 5: 32.2 fl. oz.

220 lbs./99.8 kg—Days 1 to 4: 2.64 gal | Day 5: 33.7 fl. oz.

230 lbs./104.3 kg—Days 1 to 4: 2.76 gal | Day 5: 35.3 fl. oz.

240 lbs./108.8 kg—Days 1 to 4: 2.87 gal | Day 5: 36.8 fl. oz.

250 lbs./113.4 kg—Days 1 to 4: 3.00 gal | Day 5: 38.3 fl. oz.

260 lbs./117.9 kg—Days 1 to 4: 3.11 gal | Day 5: 40.0 fl. oz.

270 lbs./122.4 kg—Days 1 to 4: 3.23 gal | Day 5: 41.4 fl. oz.

280 lbs./127.0 kg—Days 1 to 4: 3.35 gal | Day 5: 42.9 fl. oz.

290 lbs./131.5 kg—Days 1 to 4: 3.47 gal | Day 5: 44.5 fl. oz.

Water-Loading Weight Chart (Liters [l])

120 lbs./54.4 kg—Days 1 to 4: 5.4 l | Day 5: .54 l

130 lbs./59.0 kg—Days 1 to 4: 5.9 l | Day 5: .59 l

140 lbs./63.5 kg—Days 1 to 4: 6.4 l | Day 5: .64 l

150 lbs./68.0 kg—Days 1 to 4: 6.8 l | Day 5: .68 l

160 lbs./72.6 kg—Days 1 to 4: 7.3 l | Day 5: .73 l

170 lbs./77.1 kg—Days 1 to 4: 7.7 l | Day 5: .78 l

180 lbs./81.6 kg—Days 1 to 4: 8.2 l | Day 5: .82 l

190 lbs./86.2 kg—Days 1 to 4: 8.6 l | Day 5: .86 l

200 lbs./90.7 kg—Days 1 to 4: 9.1 l | Day 5: .91 l

210 lbs./95.2 kg—Days 1 to 4: 9.5 l | Day 5: .95 l

220 lbs./99.8 kg—Days 1 to 4: 10.0 l | Day 5: 1.0 l

230 lbs./104.3 kg—Days 1 to 4: 10.4 l | Day 5: 1.04 l
240 lbs./108.8 kg—Days 1 to 4: 10.9 l | Day 5: 1.09 l
250 lbs./113.4 kg—Days 1 to 4: 11.3 l | Day 5: 1.13 l
260 lbs./117.9 kg—Days 1 to 4: 11.8 l | Day 5: 1.18 l
270 lbs./122.4 kg—Days 1 to 4: 12.2 l | Day 5: 1.22 l
280 lbs./127.0 kg—Days 1 to 4: 12.7 l | Day 5: 1.27 l
290 lbs./131.5 kg—Days 1 to 4: 13.2 l | Day 5: 1.32 l

5. SODIUM RESTRICTION

Restricting sodium intake is another method you can use to lose body weight in the short term. Excess sodium can cause water retention, while the absence of sodium can cause water loss. Sodium is expelled from the body mainly through urination but also through perspiration. Humans can adapt to the changes in sodium balance fairly well, so results may vary from individual to individual. You may lose more or less weight, compared to someone else doing the exact same thing. When restricting sodium, avoid sports drinks, condiments, processed/packaged foods, and anything else that has a high sodium content. If you use this method, be sure to replenish sodium immediately after weighing in.

Sodium-Restriction Protocol

Do not add salt to food; consume less than 500 mg of sodium per day for 3 days before your weigh-in day. It is not necessary—and virtually impossible to—completely eliminate sodium from your diet.

6. DEHYDRATION

When it comes to making weight, dehydration typically refers to sweating and fluid restriction. The final portion of the weight cut involves sweating off the remaining weight. This is done by way of active and/or passive dehydration. In the late stages, fluid restriction or limiting water intake is also an important part of this. "Dehydration" is defined as a deficit in total body water, where more water is lost than is being taken into the body. Many of the other techniques used in this system will cause dehydration over time (a few days), but active and passive dehydration will cause immediate and rapid body-water loss. These methods can be fatiguing, so follow percentage guidelines, and stay mentally resilient throughout the process. Sweating methods should be done as close to the actual weigh-in as possible, so that athletes do not stay in a dehydrated state for an extended period. Leave room for error and time for any unforeseen issues. Some athletes begin active and/or passive dehydration the afternoon/evening before weigh-in and finish in the morning. Others prefer to do everything the morning of the weigh-in. Athlete preferences should take precedence here.

Although athletes have done this in the past, do not attempt to lose more than 5% body weight through sweating. Doing so can jeopardize health and negatively affect performance.

The body loses water through the following processes:

Urination (peeing)
Defecation (pooping)
Respiration (breathing)
Expectoration (spitting)
Perspiration (sweating)
Fluid Restriction

Sweating and **Fluid Restriction** are processes that can be controlled. The average human being can sweat off between 1.5 and 3 pounds in an hour. Men generally sweat more than women, younger individuals sweat more than older individuals, and larger individuals sweat more than smaller individuals. Fitness level also affects sweat rate; those who are more fit tend to sweat more than those who are less fit. As fitness level goes up, the body adapts and becomes more efficient at cooling down. Thus, the sweat rate increases as fitness level increases. *Thermoregulation* is the ability to maintain core body temperature. Core temperature rises in the body when the surrounding temperature is higher than skin temperature. Physical activity and exercise also cause core temperature to rise; when core temperature rises, thermoregulation kicks in to regulate body temperature. This happens by way of sweating or, more accurately, through a process known as vaporization, which is the evaporation of sweat and other bodily fluids. During intense physical activity, evaporation of sweat is responsible for much of the heat loss required to maintain core body temperature. Sweating can be active and/or passive and requires an increase in body temperature (hyperthermia). All methods of sweating can cause fatigue, so plan accordingly, and always have at least one other individual monitoring the athlete using sweating methods.

Active dehydration is done using exercise and can be paired with a passive method such as wearing additional layers or increasing room temperature to increase the sweat rate. Active dehydration will likely cause glycogen loss in addition to sweat loss, which helps with overall weight loss.

Passive dehydration involves increasing the temperature of the environment using a hot bath, sauna, or heater, or wearing layers/sauna suit. Depending on the situation or preference, some athletes use a combination of the above.

SWEATING METHODS

A. Hot Bath (Passive)

Using a hot bath is one option for increasing core temperature and getting the body to sweat quickly. Thermoregulation is affected by humidity. Under humid conditions, sweat evaporation and heat loss are limited. A hot bath allows the body to reach sufficient core temperature quicker than other methods. The temperature of the water does not need to be scalding but must be above core temperature. On average, this is 98.6°F or

37°C. Anything above 100°F (37.8°C) is hot enough for most people to trigger a sweat response. Experiment between 100°F (37.8°C) and 106°F (41.1°C). Those who are heat acclimated will be able to tolerate higher temperatures. Higher temperatures will increase sweat rate and decrease overall time but may cause increased discomfort. When limited on time, use higher temperatures. Be careful going past 108°F or 42.2°C.

Also, never be alone; carefully use assistance when exiting the bath to avoid slips and falls. Avoid fast movements as well as standing up too quickly. Doing so can cause low blood pressure and result in dizziness, light-headedness, and even a loss of consciousness. In most cases, do not exceed more than 10- to 20-minute intervals, with the first round being the longest and the subsequent rounds shorter. Do not attempt to lose more than 5% of your body weight using any sweating method, as doing so can jeopardize health and negatively impact performance.

The second part of any sweating method is to fully cover the body with a sauna suit/layers/blankets/towels immediately after each session to trap heat and continue the sweating process until sweating stops. Put an ice bag or a cold towel on your forehead, and monitor your forehead to know when sweating has stopped. Monitor overheating, and remove your arms from the wrap if the heat becomes uncomfortable. This process lasts around 30 to 40 minutes and is typically called the "burrito." Take long-enough breaks between rounds to allow for the body to cool down and reset (typically 20 to 30 minutes). Once you are cooled down, dry off completely, and check weight. Repeat if necessary.

B. INFRARED SAUNA (PASSIVE)

Some athletes prefer using a sauna to dehydrate. A portable or non-portable infrared sauna is also a solid option. Infrared saunas do not tax the respiratory system as much as traditional dry saunas. Do not exceed more than 20- to 30-minute intervals, with the first round being the longest and the subsequent rounds shorter. Do not attempt to lose more than 5% of your body weight using any sweating method, as doing so can jeopardize health and negatively impact performance.

Then, as with any sweating method, fully cover the body with a sauna suit/layers/blankets/towels immediately after each session to trap heat and continue the sweating process until sweating stops. Put an ice bag or a cold towel on your forehead, and monitor your forehead to know when sweating has stopped. Monitor overheating, and remove your arms from the wrap if the heat becomes uncomfortable. This process lasts around 30 to 40 minutes, and is typically called the "burrito". Take long-enough breaks between rounds to allow for the body to cool down and reset (typically 20 to 30 minutes). Once you are cooled down, dry off completely, and check weight. Repeat if necessary.

C. TRADITIONAL DRY SAUNA (PASSIVE OR PASSIVE AND ACTIVE)

Using a traditional dry sauna is a good option for combining passive and active sweating methods. For example, combining light cardio or shadowboxing with heat stress increases your sweat rate and decreases the time it takes to begin sweating. This can decrease the overall time you spend making weight. However, using a traditional dry sauna can tax the respiratory system. For this reason, it is more effective to use a traditional dry sauna for shorter durations and when cutting smaller amounts of weight. Do not exceed more than 10- to 20-minute intervals, with the first round being the longest and the subsequent rounds shorter. Do not attempt to lose more than 5% of your body weight using any sweating method, as doing so can jeopardize health and negatively impact performance.

Then, as with any sweating method, fully cover the body with a sauna suit/layers/blankets/towels immediately after each session to trap heat and continue the sweating process until sweating stops. Put an ice bag or a cold towel on your forehead, and monitor your forehead to know when sweating has stopped. Monitor overheating, and remove your arms from the wrap if the heat becomes uncomfortable. This process lasts around 30 to 40 minutes, and is typically called the "burrito". Take long-enough breaks between rounds to allow for the body to cool down and reset (typically 20 to 30 minutes). Once you are cooled down, dry off completely, and check weight. Repeat if necessary.

D. EXERCISE (ACTIVE OR ACTIVE AND PASSIVE)

Any type of exercise done continuously and with enough intensity will raise core temperature and cause sweating.

Active sweating methods can include running, shadowboxing, cardio machines, biking, body-weight movements, drilling, bag/pad work, grappling, circuit training, etc. Active sweating methods can be combined with a passive method by using a heated environment or by wearing additional layers. Do not attempt to lose more than 5% of your body weight using this method. Remember that active dehydration will likely cause glycogen loss in addition to sweat loss. This helps with overall weight loss but can cause fatigue. Be cautious and do not to get overly fatigued using active-dehydration methods. Once the core temperature has risen and your body is sweating at a sufficient rate, move on to part two. Conserve your energy.

Then, as with any sweating method, fully cover the body with a sauna suit/layers/blankets/towels immediately after each session to trap heat and continue the sweating process until sweating stops. Put an ice bag or a cold towel on your forehead, and monitor your forehead to know when sweating has stopped. Monitor overheating, and remove your arms from the wrap if the heat becomes uncomfortable. This process lasts around 30 to 40 minutes, and is typically called the "burrito". Take long-enough breaks between rounds to allow for the body to cool down and reset (typically 20 to 30 minutes). Once you are cooled down, dry off completely, and check weight. Repeat if necessary.

Fluid Restriction

Limiting fluids in the last 24 to 36 hours before weigh-in will further dehydrate the body and contribute to weight loss. This includes eliminating foods that have a high fluid content, such as fruits and food that is steamed or boiled.

SWEATING-SESSION EXAMPLES

A. Passive Only

1. Sit comfortably in a hot bath or sauna for 10 to 20 minutes. This duration can be longer if an athlete is heat acclimated.
2. Exit carefully, and use assistance. Avoid fast movements and standing up too quickly.
3. Immediately cover your body with sauna suit/layers/blankets/towels to trap heat and continue sweating.
4. Put an ice bag or a cold towel on your forehead, and relax. Monitor your forehead for beads of sweat.
5. Once sweating has stopped, take a break to allow your body to cool down and prevent overheating. Once dry, check your weight. Repeat as needed.

B. Active Only

1. Perform any continuous low-intensity exercise, such as shadowboxing, running, biking, body-weight movements, drilling, pad work, grappling, circuit training, cardio machines, etc.
2. The goal is to build up a good sweat and increase core body temperature while keeping your fatigue level low. Building up a good sweat can take anywhere from 15 to 45 minutes, depending on the individual.

3. Fully cover your body with sauna suit/layers/blankets/ towels to trap heat and continue sweating.

4. Put an ice bag or a cold towel on your forehead and relax. Monitor forehead for beads of sweat.

5. Once sweating has stopped, take a break to allow your body to cool down and prevent overheating. Once dry, check your weight. Repeat as needed.

C. Active and Passive

1. Wear additional layers or a sauna suit—or use a heated room or sauna.

2. Perform any continuous, low-intensity exercise such as shadowboxing, running, biking, body-weight movements, drilling, pad work, grappling, circuit training, cardio machines, etc.

3. Fully cover your body with sauna suit/layers/blankets/ towels to trap heat and continue sweating.

4. Put an ice bag or a cold towel on your forehead, and relax. Monitor your forehead for beads of sweat.

5. Once sweating has stopped, take a break to allow your body to cool down and prevent overheating. Once dry, check your weight. Repeat as needed.

7. PHASE 3: POST-WEIGH-IN

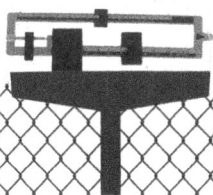

O nce weigh-ins are complete, your goal is to replenish what was taken out of the body. Immediately upon stepping off the official scale, focus on getting to the competition well hydrated, with optimal electrolytes, and with replenished glycogen stores. Avoid consuming anything that can be detrimental to performance, such as high-fat and high-fiber foods. Avoid consuming foods with which you are unfamiliar.

After the weigh-in, you want your first drink to be hypotonic (containing less than 6% carbohydrate content). Hypotonic solutions are absorbed faster by the body than isotonic (6–8% carbohydrate content) and hypertonic (+10% carbohydrate content) solutions. This comes down to gastric emptying, or how quickly fluid is moved into the small intestine. Most oral rehydration solutions are hypotonic, while most sports drinks are isotonic, and most energy drinks are hypertonic. After replenishing fluids and electrolytes, replenish carbohydrates and then food.

POST WEIGH-IN

1. Replenish fluids and electrolytes
2. Replenish carbohydrates
3. Consume low-fat and low-fiber foods
4. Monitor hydration
5. Supplements (optional)

REPLENISH FLUIDS AND ELECTROLYTES

Replenish fluids and electrolytes as quickly as possible without causing gastrointestinal distress. In an ideal situation, you would consume 2 times the amount of weight lost during the final dehydration session. For example, if an athlete lost 6 pounds during the last dehydration session, they would consume 12 pounds of fluids, or roughly 5.5 liters over time, in addition to daily fluid requirements.

A practical guideline is 1 to 1.5 liters of fluids per hour (34 to 50 fl. oz.). Consuming fluids with added sodium and carbohydrates can speed up the rehydration process. During exercise, your body primarily loses sodium, also a small amount of potassium, and a tiny amount of calcium.

Electrolytes are a subgroup of minerals that have many functions, including helping the body absorb water and maintaining homeostasis. Electrolytes include sodium, potassium, calcium, and magnesium. Most individuals are able to ingest 1 liter or 33.8 oz. of water per hour without issues, but some athletes may find it difficult to drink fluids in a dehydrated state without electrolytes. Be sure to add electrolytes, or use an oral rehydration solution (ORS) immediately after weigh-in. Especially if there was heavy sweating or water restriction involved during the final dehydration. Pedialyte, Hydralyte, Drip Drop, and Gatorlytes are examples of recognized brands.

REPLENISH CARBOHYDRATES

Consume carbohydrates about 30 to 45 minutes after replenishing fluids and electrolytes. Remember to continue replenishing fluids, electrolytes, and carbohydrates until a few hours before the competition. Virtually all combat sports require anaerobic energy-system contribution. Especially when there is little time between the weigh-in and competition, glycogen depletion can negatively impact performance. Having fully replenished carbohydrate stores will benefit your performance even if you did not consume a low-carbohydrate diet or use glycogen depletion. The average human body can process around 1g of carbohydrate per minute due to the absorption rate of the intestines (60g in 1 hour). Using multiple carbohydrate sources allows the body to process closer to 90g of carbohydrates per hour. When replenishing carbohydrates, limit complex carbohydrates and excessive fiber intake. Overconsuming fiber can cause stomach discomfort after being on a low-fiber diet.

TWO TYPES OF CARBOHYDRATES:

1. Simple—sugars, usually easy to digest and provide quick energy to the body (refined grains, sports drinks).
2. Complex—higher in nutritional content; often contains fiber (greens, whole grains).

After weighing in, immediately consume fluids with electrolytes, and give your body time to rehydrate. Wait 30 to 45 minutes before consuming simple carbohydrates and a small amount of protein. For example: salted pretzels, banana, and protein shake. If you do not have time to wait because the competition is about to begin, consume the carbohydrates immediately, and skip the protein. For competitions that give you more time to recover, wait another 60 to 90 minutes before consuming a solid meal.

Use a 4:1 carbohydrate-to-protein ratio when refueling with solid meals. For example: 100g carbohydrates, 25g protein.

CONSUME LOW-FAT AND LOW-FIBER FOODS

Upon completion of weigh-ins, avoid stuffing yourself with high-calorie foods, and especially avoid consuming anything with high-fat or high-fiber content. Excessive fat or excessive fiber intake can lead to stomach discomfort as well as diminished performance. On top of that, high-fat and high-fiber foods slow down the nutrient-absorption rate. You want nutrients to get into your system as fast as possible. Be sure also to stick to foods that you're familiar with. This is not the time to be trying new things you've never had before.

MONITOR HYDRATION

Performance can suffer if you are operating in a dehydrated state. You can monitor hydration status by using a self-monitoring system called WUT (Weight, Urine, Thirst). The WUT system can also be used during camp, when you're not trying to cut weight, and requires only a body-weight scale.

WUT SYSTEM

1. **Weight (W)**—Use bathroom first thing in the morning, and weigh yourself naked before eating or drinking. Record this weight, and keep a log. A loss of more than 1% of your average morning body weight is an indicator of dehydration.

Did you lose more than 1% of your body weight? (YES/NO)

2. **Urine (U)**—The body produces less urine when sweat loss is high and the amount of water in the body is low. When less urine is produced, it can become darker and more concentrated. Use the color of apple juice or darker as a guide. Optimal urine color is the color of lemonade (colorless urine could be an indicator of over-hydration). Dark-colored urine is another indicator of dehydration.

Is your urine as dark or darker than apple juice? (YES/NO)

3. **Thirst (T)**—Thirst is the body telling you to drink fluids. Thirst can develop after you are already dehydrated, and not being thirsty does not mean that you are not dehydrated. Thirst is another indicator of dehydration.

Are feeling thirsty? (YES/NO)

Results: If you answered YES to 2 or more of the questions above, it is likely that you are in a dehydrated state.

Having 2 indicators present means you are likely dehydrated. Having all 3 indicators present means you are very likely dehydrated.

SUPPLEMENTS

Glutamine and caffeine supplementation can also aid rehydration, but take caution when using supplements. Especially supplements which you are unfamiliar with. Only ingest supplements that have been tested for banned substances and have been certified by organizations such as "NSF" or "Informed Sport."

POST WEIGH-IN PROTOCOL

1. Immediately upon making weight: Rehydrate by drinking .5 to 1 liter (16.9 to 33.8 fl. oz) of fluids containing at least one full serving of an ORS (oral rehydration solution).

For example, Pedialyte, Liquid IV, Drip Drop, Hydralyte, Gatorlytes, etc. Larger athletes may need 1.5 to 2 full servings. Temporary stomach discomfort can be avoided by drinking slowly, but it's important to quickly get the body out of a dehydrated state.

2. After rehydrating, wait 30 to 45 minutes and consume a mostly liquid meal consisting of mostly carbohydrates. Consume 60 to 90 grams of carbohydrates, and ideally use two different forms of carbs for more rapid absorption. Use a 2:1 ratio of Glucose or Dextrose to Fructose. You may also consume some protein if the competition is not immediately following weigh-in.

EXAMPLES:

A. 2–3 Packs Energy Gel, 8 oz. Cold Pressed Juice
B. Salted Pretzels, Banana, Protein Shake
C. Cereal and Milk

* If the competition is immediately following weigh-in or less than 2 hours after weigh-in, do not wait, and combine steps 1 and 2. Skip step 3 and step 4.

3. After consuming a liquid meal, wait another 60 to 90 minutes before consuming a solid meal high in carbohydrates, low in fiber, and low in fat. A 4:1 carbohydrate-to-protein ratio is a good place to start when refueling with solid meals. Aim for 80–120g of carbohydrates with 20–30g of protein.

4. Monitor hydration status by using self-monitoring or other reliable forms of hydration testing. Drink 34–50 oz. of water per hour. Stop 3–4 hours before bed and before the competition. Continue to consume solid meals every 3–5 hours that are high in carbohydrates, low in fiber, and low in fat.

   * If you walk around on weight and did not use any dehydration methods for making weight, then simply ensure that your carbohydrate stores are replenished, monitor hydration status, and stick to consuming familiar foods.

8. GUIDES

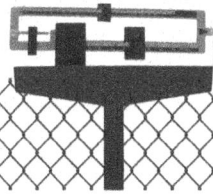

PROFESSIONAL MMA ATHLETE

In this example, the athlete has completed the Phase 1 preparation and will be competing approximately 30 to 36 hours after weigh-in.

Current Weight (5 days to weigh-in day): 183 lbs. (83.0 kg)
Weigh-in Weight (1 pound allowance): 171 lbs. (77.6 kg)

SUNDAY:
Water Loading: **2.2 gal (8.3 l)**
Heat Acclimation: **30 minutes in hot tub or sauna**

*Consume meals that are familiar to you

MONDAY:
Water Loading: **2.2 gal (8.3 l)**
Heat Acclimation: **30 minutes in hot tub or sauna**

*Consume meals that are familiar to you

TUESDAY:
Gut Content Elimination: **<5g fiber**
Glycogen Depletion: **<50g carbohydrates**
Water Loading: **2.2 gal (8.3 l)**
Sodium Restriction: **<500 mg sodium**
Heat Acclimation: **Rest day**

   *Consume meals that are familiar to you: low in fiber, fat, carbohydrates, and sodium

WEDNESDAY:
Gut-Content Elimination: **<5g fiber**
Glycogen Depletion: **<50g carbohydrates**
Water Loading: **2.2 gal (8.3 l)**
Sodium Restriction: **<500 mg sodium**
Heat Acclimation: **30 minutes in hot tub or sauna**

   *Consume meals that are familiar to you: low in fiber, fat, carbohydrates, and sodium

THURSDAY (Water restriction day):
Gut-Content Elimination: **<5g fiber**
Glycogen Depletion: **<50g carbohydrates**
Water Restriction: **No more than 28 fl. oz. (0.83 l)**
Sodium Restriction: **<500 mg sodium**

   *Stop drinking fluids in the afternoon
   *Consume meals that are familiar to you: low in fiber, fat, carbohydrates, and sodium

*Active/Passive dehydration protocol can be done on this day in the afternoon/evening for athletes who prefer to cut some or all of the weight the night before weigh-in.

FRIDAY (Weigh-In 9 a.m. to 11 a.m.):
5:00 a.m.—Wake up
5:30 a.m.—Begin "Active/Passive Dehydration Protocol"
9:00 a.m.—Official weigh-in
9:15 a.m.—Begin "Post-Weigh-In Protocol": Drink half a bottle of Pedialyte; fill other half with water, and finish
10:00 a.m.—Mostly liquid meal: Salted pretzels, banana, protein shake

*Drink 34 to 50 fl. oz. of fluids *per hour* until 3–4 hours before bed to avoid sleep disturbance. Continue the following day, and stop drinking 3–4 hours before competition. Take sips as needed. Avoid high-fat, high-fiber foods.

11:30 a.m.—Lean steak, pasta with red sauce
3:00 p.m.—Chicken sandwich on white bread, baked chips
7:00 p.m.—Salmon, white rice, canned spinach
10:00 p.m.—Protein shake, milk chocolate
1:00 a.m.—Sleep

*If mouth is dry, consume nothing until after weigh-in. Then suck on hard candy or ice chips, and spit.
*After weigh-in, use post weigh-in protocols in Phase 3.
*Continue to consume meals that are familiar to you: low in fiber and fat.

SATURDAY (Competition 7:30 p.m.):
10:00 a.m.—Wake up
10:30 a.m.—Oatmeal or grits, Omelet: eggs/bacon/tomatoes, orange juice or any juice not containing high amounts of fiber
1:30 p.m.—Chicken breast, white rice, canned beets, or fruit
4:30 p.m.—White bread, banana, honey, 24oz of Gatorade
6:55 p.m.—Handful of jelly beans or gummy candy
7:30 p.m.—Walkout

*Continue to consume meals that are familiar to you: low in fiber and fat

AMATEUR MMA ATHLETE

In this example, the athlete has completed the Phase 1 preparation and will be competing approximately 10 hours after weigh-in. Because there is less time to replenish glycogen stores, you will not restrict carbohydrates and instead focus on the other main protocols. If there is a large amount of weight that must be lost, you may have to restrict carbohydrates, depending on the situation.

Current Weight (5 days to weigh-in day): 177 lbs. (80.0 kg)
Weigh-in Weight (1 lb. allowance): 171 lbs. (77.6 kg)

MONDAY:
Water Loading: **2.1 gal (8.0 l)**
Heat Acclimation: **20 minutes in hot tub or sauna**

*Consume meals that are familiar to you

TUESDAY:

Water Loading: **2.1 gal (8.0 l)**

Heat Acclimation: **20 minutes in hot tub or sauna**

*Consume meals that are familiar to you

WEDNESDAY:

Water Loading: **2.1 gal (8.0 l)**

Gut-Content Elimination: **<5g fiber**

Sodium Restriction: **<500 mg sodium**

Heat Acclimation: **Rest day**

*Consume meals that are familiar to you: low in fiber, fat, and sodium

THURSDAY:

Water Loading: **2.1 gal (8.0 l)**

Gut-Content Elimination: **<5g fiber**

Sodium Restriction: **<500 mg sodium**

Heat Acclimation: **20 minutes in hot tub or sauna**

*Consume meals that are familiar to you: low in fiber, fat, and sodium

FRIDAY (Water Restriction):

Water Loading: **No more than 28 fl. oz. (0.80 l)**

Gut-Content Elimination: **<5g fiber**

Sodium Restriction: **<500 mg sodium**

*Stop drinking fluids in the afternoon.

*Consume meals that are familiar to you: low in fiber, fat, and sodium.

*Active/Passive dehydration protocol can be done on this day in the afternoon/evening for athletes who prefer to cut some or all of the weight the night before weigh-in.

SATURDAY (Weigh-in 8 a.m. to 9 a.m., Competition 6 p.m.):
4:30 a.m.—Wake up
5:00 a.m.—Begin "Active/Passive Dehydration Protocol"
8:00 a.m.—Official weigh-in
8:35 a.m.—Begin "Post-Weigh-in Protocol": Drink 2 full servings of an ORS, such as DripDrop mixed with 32 oz. water
9:00 a.m.—Mostly liquid meal: Cereal and milk, 8–12 oz. cold pressed juice

*Drink 34 to 50 fl. oz. of fluids *per hour* until 3–4 hours before before competition. Then take sips as needed. Avoid high-fat, high-fiber foods.

11:30 p.m.—Salmon, white rice, banana
12:15 p.m.—Nap
2:30 p.m.—Chicken breast, white rice, small sports drink
5:30 p.m.—Handful of jelly beans or gummy candy
6:00 p.m.—Walkout

AMATEUR JIU-JITSU ATHLETE

In this example, the athlete has done the proper Phase 1 preparation and will be competing approximately 30 minutes to 1 hour after weigh-in. Because there is much less time to replenish glycogen and electrolytes, you will not restrict carbohydrates or sodium, and instead focus on the other main protocols.

Current Weight (5 days to weigh-in day): 172 lbs. (78.0 kg)
Weigh-in Weight (no allowance): 168 lbs. (76.1 kg)

MONDAY:
Water Loading: **2.0 gal (7.8 l)**

  *Consume meals that are familiar to you

TUESDAY:
Water Loading: **2.0 gal (7.8 l)**

  *Consume meals that are familiar to you

WEDNESDAY:
Water Loading: **2.0 gal (7.8 l)**
Gut-Content Elimination: **<5g fiber**

  *Consume meals that are familiar to you: low in fiber and fat

THURSDAY:
Water Loading: **2.0 gal (7.8 l)**
Gut-Content Elimination: **<5g fiber**

   *Consume meals that are familiar to you: low in fiber and fat

FRIDAY:
Water Loading: **No more than 26 fl. oz. (0.78 l)**
Gut-Content Elimination: **<5g fiber**

   *Stop drinking fluids in the afternoon
   *Consume meals that are familiar to you: low in fiber and fat
   *Active/Passive dehydration protocol can be done on this day in the afternoon/evening for athletes who prefer to cut some or all of the weight the night before weigh-in

SATURDAY (Weigh-in 1 p.m., Competition 1:30 p.m.):
9:00 a.m.—Wake up
10:00 a.m.—Begin "Active/Passive Dehydration Protocol"(if needed)
1:00 p.m.—Official weigh-in (Weigh in early, if possible; this gives you more recovery time)
1:05 p.m.—Begin "Post-Weigh-in Protocol": Drink 1 full serving of an ORS such as Liquid IV, mixed with water.
   (Do not over-consume fluids at this point)

1:10 p.m.—1 to 2 energy gels, 6–8-fl. oz. cold pressed juice
1:30 p.m.—Walkout

*If there are multiple matches in one day: Monitor hydration, and continue to rehydrate between matches. Consume 30g to 60g of simple carbohydrates about half an hour before each match. Avoid high-fat and high-fiber foods.

9. DANGERS OF WEIGHT CUTTING

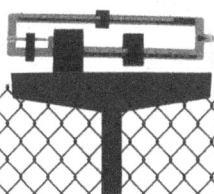

When competing in a sport with weight classes, the purpose of cutting weight is to allow an athlete to get down to a lower weight class. In a match, the athlete tends to have a competitive advantage. Gaining a competitive advantage is beneficial, but should not be prioritized over arriving to the competition well-hydrated, and with adequate carbohydrate intake. Risk versus reward must be considered on an individual basis when it comes to weight cutting.

For example, let's say you're a professional MMA athlete competing in the UFC or a professional grappler competing in ADCC. You will most likely have to cut weight in order to be competitive unless you are in the heaviest weight-class. The higher the level of competition, the more optimized your weight-cutting strategy must be. On the flip side, if you're a novice jiu-jitsu student competing in your first tournament, cutting weight most likely isn't worth the risk and additional stress.

The athlete cutting weight must be monitored by a professional for increased heart rate and decreased blood pressure.

Having a pulse oximeter and a blood pressure cuff on hand is essential. Here are some of the things to look for with regards to safety. Remember: This is not medical advice.

ORTHOSTATIC HYPOTENSION

Fast movements and rapidly standing up can cause low blood pressure, which can result in dizziness and light-headedness. Athletes can pass out from this. Be careful, and use assistance at all times, especially when exiting a sauna or hot bath.

LOW ENERGY

Being in a caloric deficit can impact your performance during training. Carbohydrates are the primary source of energy for high-intensity exercise, and protein/amino acids are the building blocks for repair. When your body is lacking calories, your endocrine system and hormone balance will be affected. Your immune system can become compromised, which makes you more susceptible to illness and/or injury.

DEHYDRATION (MEDICAL CONDITION)

Dehydration, as a medical condition, occurs when water loss becomes greater than water intake. Over time, this leads to a deficit in total body water. Dehydration causes the body's temperature to rise, increases risk for electrolyte loss, elevates heart rate, and, in the extreme, can cause heatstroke, heart failure, or kidney damage. A decrease in performance can be seen at around 2% dehydration. Most individuals experience a massive decrease in performance and begin feeling extreme fatigue and dizziness at around 5% dehydration. Electrolyte imbalance, as a result of dehydration, can also cause the muscles to fire inefficiently, increasing the risk of injury.

Dehydration affects performance by negatively impacting aerobic endurance, aerobic capacity, and heat tolerance. Strength and power are also negatively affected but to a lesser degree. A 2% or more loss of fluids during exercise can occur in as quickly as 60–90 minutes, depending on factors such as body size, exercise intensity, environment, and clothing. Individual tolerance to dehydration can also vary, and your sweat rate decreases in colder environments. In colder environments, the air around the skin is cooler, which allows for more heat loss to occur before sweating. This is why it takes longer to sweat in colder environments, where you must increase your core temperature and build up a sweat before heat loss can occur via evaporation.

For a 68-kg or 150-lb. individual, a 2% loss of fluids equates to about 1.5 l or 3.3 lbs. of sweat.

Athletes who go thorough intense weight cuts can become fatigued or "gas out" earlier in fights due to dehydration. Athletes competing in a dehydrated state may have less ability to absorb strikes to the head. It is known that dehydration can affect performance, but it can also affect the brain. In combat sports, you need to use your brain during competition. You need to think, apply strategy, and problem-solve in real-time.

Being compromised in this department is not an effective long-term strategy.

EFFECTS OF DEHYDRATION AND BODY-WATER LOSS:

.5%—Increased cardiac stress (> cardiac output, heart rate)
1%—Decreased aerobic endurance
2%—Reduced blood flow to brain (< cognitive function)
3%—Decreased muscular endurance
4%—Decreased muscular strength and motor skills
5%—Heat exhaustion (severe fatigue)

SIGNS AND SYMPTOMS OF SEVERE DEHYDRATION:

Tachycardia (RHR >100–120bpm or drastically above baseline)
Dizziness
Headache
Sunken eyes
Skin elasticity (skin takes more time to return to normal position when pinched, clammy skin)
Severe cognitive impairment

ELECTROLYTE LOSS

Electrolytes conduct an electrical current in water, regulate blood pressure, regulate heart rate, transmit nerve impulses, and are responsible for muscle contraction. For optimal performance, electrolytes lost during the weight-making process must be replenished.

Electrolytes include:

Sodium (Na)
Potassium (K)
Magnesium (Mg)
Calcium (Ca)
Chloride (Cl)
Phosphate (P)
Bicarbonate (HCO)

Sodium and calcium are utilized for muscular contraction. Potassium is utilized for muscular relaxation, and magnesium regulates the other electrolytes going into and out of the cell. When these substances in the body become imbalanced, it can lead to either muscle weakness or excessive contraction and cramping.

HYPONATREMIA

The electrolyte-deficiency disorder known as hyponatremia is one of the biggest risk factors when it comes to weight cutting. Hyponatremia happens when there is low sodium concentration in the blood. Over-hydration, or drinking too much water without electrolytes, in a short amount of time, can cause hyponatremia. Water intoxication happens when water intake is beyond the kidney's ability to filter it. Make sure to monitor water loading, and drink no more than 50 oz. of fluids per hour.

HYPOVOLEMIA

Another risk factor associated with dehydration is a decrease in blood-plasma volume, known as hypovolemia. Blood plasma is the pale-yellow-liquid portion of blood, minus the red blood cells, white blood cells, and platelets. Blood plasma carries nutrients, hormones, enzymes, and cells throughout the body, maintains normal blood pressure, and helps with heat distribution. Low blood-plasma volume causes low blood pressure and can increase risks associated with dehydration. Athletes who use laxatives or diuretics are at an increased risk of hypovolemia. If any severe symptoms arise, stop the weight cut immediately, and see a physician.

SEVERE SIGNS AND SYMPTOMS OF HYPOVOLEMIC SHOCK:

Very low urine output
Blue/purple discoloration of the fingers, toes, lips, or tongue
Hypotension (low blood pressure)
Tachycardia (resting heart rate one 100 bpm)
Mental confusion

FAT ADAPTATION

When fat is increasingly used for fuel, the body shifts toward being "fat-adapted." A diet that is high in fat and low in carbohydrates can cause this. The most common example comes from the keto diet, where the body shifts to favoring fat as the primary source of fuel. This transition can happen within a week.

Combat-sports competitions rely heavily on anaerobic contribution, and carbohydrates are the preferred source of fuel for the anaerobic energy system. Becoming "fat-adapted" during competition or during camp does not benefit performance, since compromising the body's ability to break down glycogen will not benefit high-intensity exercise. In most combat-sports competitions, explosive bursts of energy are required for scrambles or fight-ending combinations. Deciding to restrict carbohydrates can negatively affect performance. Most athletes will need carbohydrates for live sparring or intensive strength and conditioning sessions.

Athletes who get extremely overweight in between training camps and athletes who agree to competitions on short notice must often resort to low-carbohydrate diets, where there is no time for a steady decrease of caloric intake. When a low-carbohydrate diet cannot be avoided, fat adaptation can still be avoided by utilizing a high-protein diet and keeping fat intake at normal ranges.

10. EXTREME METHODS

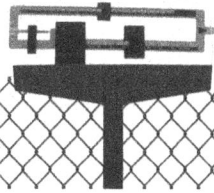

Previously, you saw charts outlining the general ranges for safely making weight. If you are not within that, reconsider accepting the bout. The following is for educational purposes. There are always outliers and talented individuals who can endure extreme weight cuts. That does not mean you should do it. Consider the risks outlined in the "Dangers of Weight Cutting" chapter.

EXTREME METHODS

1. Prolonged Glycogen Depletion
2. Fasting

PROLONGED GLYCOGEN DEPLETION

It is generally not recommended for combat-sports athletes to use a low-carbohydrate diet for longer than 3 to 5 days. Drastically decreasing carbohydrate intake over time can be detrimental to performance—especially in a sport like

MMA or any combat sport requiring bursts of high-intensity anaerobic energy.

Carbohydrates are the primary source of fuel for high-intensity energy production, and consuming fewer than 50g per day for longer than 3 to 4 days can negatively affect performance. Prolonged glycogen depletion will, however, result in even greater losses of water in the body. This is done in situations where an athlete is extremely overweight.

FASTING

Fasting essentially combines both gut-content elimination and glycogen depletion. There are athletes who regularly make weight by fasting, however, this tends to come from either a lack of knowledge or a lack of time. Since fasting is generally not optimal for performance, it is best done as close to weigh-in as possible and only when there are no other options.

Fasting can be done in many ways. For example, using intermittent fasting, you will consume calories only during a short window of time and fast for the remainder of the day. Another way is to consume calories only around training, when energy is needed. The most extreme would be to consume nothing except water—and then eliminate water in the last 12 to 24 hours before weigh-in.

11. FOODS LIST

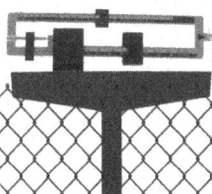

This list of foods is for the final phase of making weight. Depending on your situation, this can be around 3 to 10 days out from weigh-in. This list is meant to provide examples so that you can apply your own personal preferences. It is not a complete list of all possible options. Experiment in the off-season, or far in advance of competition, to ensure that there are no unexpected outcomes. Making weight for competition isn't about maximizing health benefits, but it is still important to avoid dangerous and prolonged methods that can lead to detrimental long-term health effects. When not in the final phase of making weight, focus on maintaining a caloric deficit, with the goal of getting relatively lean.

You do not need to stick to this list until the last few days before weigh-in. Consume foods that are low in fiber, low in fat, and high in energy (calories). Depending on the situation, overall daily carbohydrate intake must also be monitored. Foods that are moderate in fat can be acceptable, but avoid high-fat foods, which can be detrimental to performance. Athletes who are within the guidelines outlined earlier can transition to this list of foods 3 days out from weigh-in. Starting sooner may be necessary, depending on the amount of weight that must be lost.

In addition, during the final 24 to 36 hours before weigh-in, you want to consume more liquid meals and foods that are low in weight and volume. Once you begin fluid restriction, remember to avoid foods that contain large amounts of water. Cooking with methods that remove water, such as pan-frying, will also aid in fluid restriction during the final 24 to 36 hours. Avoid preparation methods that can add water, such as boiling, steaming, poaching, braising, and stewing.

PROTEIN

Meat and Poultry
Eggs
Beef (ground)
Beef (steak)
Chicken (ground)
Chicken (breast/thigh)
Pork (ground)
Pork (chops)
Pork (lean bacon)
Turkey (ground)
Turkey (bacon)
Salmon
Whitefish
Shrimp
Scallops

* Avoid cuts of meat with high fat content

Dairy

Protein powder

Cottage cheese, hard cheeses (cheddar, Parmesan)

Milk (2% or lower)

Plain Yogurt (2% or lower)

* Avoid dairy products with high fat content

CARBOHYDRATES

Vegetables

Any canned vegetables with low-fiber

Canned beets

Canned spinach

Canned tomatoes

Canned asparagus

Canned green beans

Canned carrots

Baby food

Potatoes (no skin)

Vegetable juice (no pulp)

Tomato sauce

* Avoid all vegetables with high fiber content

* Avoid raw/cruciferous vegetables

* Avoid beans and lentils

* Avoid skin and peels of vegetables

Grains
White bread
White crackers
White rice
Rice cakes
Low-fiber cereal
Grits

* Avoid all grains with high fiber content
* Avoid whole grains, wild/brown rice

Fruits
Any canned fruits with low fiber
Canned beets
Canned mandarin oranges
Canned peaches
Baby food
Applesauce
Bananas
Cantaloupe
Honeydew
Watermelon
Jam/jelly with no seeds
Fruit juice (no pulp)

* Avoid all fruits with high-fiber content
* Avoid skin and peels of fruit
* Avoid raw or dried fruits

Other Carbohydrates
Milk chocolate
Energy gels
Jelly beans
Gummy candy
Fruit chews

   * Avoid anything with high-fiber or high-fat content
   * If using glycogen depletion, moderate and even high-carb foods can be consumed before training, as long as overall daily carbohydrate intake is monitored and below threshold.

FATS

Butter
Ghee
Olive oil
Corn oil
Peanut oil
Coconut oil
Avocado oil
Grape-seed oil
Canola oil
Safflower oil
Mayonnaise
Cashew butter

   * Avoid anything with high-fat content
   * Avoid nuts and seeds that are not in oil form

EXAMPLES

Example 1
* 3 days out from weigh-in
* Avoid anything with high-fat and high-fiber content

Meal 1: Hard-boiled eggs, turkey bacon, grits, coffee
Meal 2: Ground beef, low-fiber vegetables, white rice
Meal 3: PB&J sandwich on white bread, protein shake
Meal 4: Meatballs, canned tomatoes, pasta
Meal 5: Salmon with butter and lemon, white rice, protein shake

Example 2
* 24 hours out from weigh-in
* Avoid anything with high-fat or high-fiber content
* Fluid restriction
* Sodium restriction

Meal 1: Pan-fried eggs, white toast, coffee
Meal 2: Pan-fried ribeye steak, canned spinach, white rice
Meal 3: Chicken breast or thigh, canned tomatoes, white rice
Meal 4: Milk chocolate, protein shake
Meal 5: Cottage cheese, canned oranges, protein pudding

12. FAQ

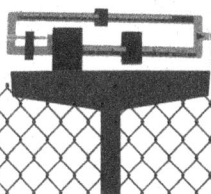

20. Jetlag
21. Altitude
22. Mental

1. RED FLAGS

Cutting weight for competition is not for average people. It takes an individual who can handle the physical and mental challenges involved with the process. Safety must always be prioritized. To understand the consequences, refer to the chapter on the dangers of weight cutting.

If an athlete shows any of the following signs, immediately stop and consult with a physician:

- Panic
- Sharp increase in resting heart rate/Sharp increase in resting heart rate
- Clamminess in skin
- Severe cognitive impairment

2. DIFFERENCES IN MEN AND WOMEN

The menstrual cycle for women can cause hormonal changes that lead to increased water retention and weight gain. Some women choose to take birth-control medication to prevent this. Generally speaking, women have higher body fat and lower muscle mass than men. Since muscle is where the majority of water is held, women tend to sweat less than men and have less potential to lose water. Women also tend to sweat less than men, so it may take longer for women to cut the same amount of weight. This does not apply to all women, especially when it comes to elite, highly trained, and extremely lean female athletes.

3. DISTILLED WATER

Distilled water tends to pass through the body directly into the bladder. This increases urine output and can lead to electrolyte imbalances—particularly in sodium, calcium, and potassium. Distilled water is often used to beat a hydration test. It does not need to be used when cutting weight.

4. HYDRATION TESTING

The most common hydration test in combat sports is urine osmolality or urine-specific gravity testing. The normal range for urine-specific gravity is 1.005 to 1.030. Some organizations require testing at 1.025 or below, meaning that the athlete cannot be severely dehydrated.

But urine-hydration tests may not be useful at all for assessing actual hydration level, since urine in the bladder serves no function. Instead of useful information, this may lead to false positives. Even serum/plasma osmolality has potential flaws, such as human error.

Organizations that require hydration testing often deal with athletes gaming the test in order to make weight. Athletes can game hydration tests by water loading during the week and cutting 1–2 lbs. of water past the contracted weight. This is followed by chugging 1–2 lbs. of distilled water back into the body up to the weight limit. Done 30–45 minutes before weigh-in, this dilutes the athlete's urine and is a method for beating urine-based hydration tests.

5. MULTIPLE-DAY WEIGH-IN

You will not be able to cut a lot of weight when there are multiple days you must weigh in—especially if the Day-1 weight must be made on multiple consecutive days.

Competitions such as ADCC have multiple weigh-ins on 3 consecutive days.[*] In these types of competitions, your competition weight must stay around your weigh-in weight.

After weighing in on Day 1, consume foods that are low in weight and high in energy (calories). Combine this with continuing to limit fiber and sodium intake. If necessary, use active/passive dehydration methods on each day before weigh-in.

6. SUPPLEMENTS (BEFORE WEIGH-IN)

Before the weigh-in, there are two types of supplements that tend to be used.

- Ingested supplements
- Topical creams

---

[*] As of 2024, ADCC has changed to single day weigh-in. However, other competitions such as freestyle wrestling still enforce multiple-day weigh-in.

Ingested supplements such as dandelion root and celery seed are classified as diuretics. Diuretics help your kidneys release more sodium into your urine; using these supplements may slightly increase body-water loss. But this comes with a risk for adverse effects. Relying on diuretics during a weight cut is generally not an effective strategy.

Virtually all laxatives should be avoided. Laxatives can cause excessive electrolyte loss, and athletes who use them tend to feel unwell. If you must use a diuretic for constipation, a mild diuretic supplement containing Senna leaves can be used prior to bedtime, early in the week when you begin to eliminate fiber.

Topical creams such as Sweet Sweat, Albolene, or other topical creams containing petroleum jelly can increase your sweat rate when applied directly to the skin. Using these topical supplements may increase body-water loss and decrease the time it takes to start sweating. Topical creams do appear to be effective, but they are not always necessary.

7. SUPPLEMENTS (AFTER WEIGH-IN)

After the weigh-in, caffeine and glutamine can be used to aid in the rehydration process. Caffeine has been shown to increase glycogen re-synthesis. Since there is a high individual response to caffeine, an athlete who supplements with caffeine should also be consuming caffeine regularly. Glutamine can also aid with rehydration by pulling sodium and water out of the small intestine and increasing the hydration rate of the body.

8. SUPPLEMENTS (GENERAL)

General supplements such as multivitamins, probiotics, protein powders, vitamin C, vitamin D, vitamin K, magnesium, zinc, etc. can be used throughout the weight-making process. Take only supplements you are familiar with and have used throughout camp. Check nutrition labels, and avoid supplements which can interfere with the goals of the weight cut.

If you supplement with creatine, it should be removed 2–4 weeks before weigh-in. Creatine tends to cause water retention, and, by removing it, the body will hold on to less water. After the weigh-in, loading creatine can increase weight regain and possibly increase performance, depending on the athlete's individual response. If you supplement with beta alanine, continue taking 4 to 6 grams per day prior to training sessions.

9. CHECKING WEIGHT

Check weight first thing in the morning, after using the bathroom. Use the same scale, and be sure to calibrate it with the official weigh-in scale or official test scale. It is wise to invest in a high-quality shipping scale; remember to place scale on a flat surface but not on carpet or an uneven surface.

10. EPSOM SALT AND ALCOHOL

Adding epsom salt or alcohol to a hot bath does not directly increase water loss in the body. During a hot bath, water exits the body as a response to heat. Heat is the primary mechanism for increasing perspiration or sweating, which then leads to body-water loss and dehydration over time.

With that said, the mind plays a large role in all things. Adding alcohol to a hot bath can give an athlete a cooling sensation. And an athlete who perceives the water temperature as cooler than it actually is can tolerate higher temperatures. Adding epsom salt to a hot bath provides a visual stimulus that can give an athlete a psychological boost. Epsom salt also breaks down into magnesium and sulfate, which are minerals that can be depleted during the weight cut. Although transdermal absorption is not fully understood, adding these minerals back into the body can increase an athlete's overall feeling of well-being.

11. CRAMPING

Muscle cramping is sudden and involuntary muscular contractions. Cramping occurs due to a combination of:

- Electrolyte imbalance (particularly lack of sodium)
- Lack of fluids in the muscle due to being dehydrated
- Lack of glycogen in the muscle due to lack of carbohydrates

* Muscle fatigue and other neurological factors

12. ONLY DRINKING WATER AFTER WEIGH-IN

Dehydration from sweating causes the loss of both water and electrolytes. Only drinking water will lower electrolyte concentration in the body and cause excessive urination. This is not optimal for rehydration. Even if dehydration was not utilized to make weight, consuming water with carbohydrates and electrolytes will ensure that the body is replenished and ready for competition.

13. MINORS AND WEIGHT CUTTING

Weight cutting should not be encouraged with younger athletes. Young athletes are still growing, and their bodies are going through changes. Not having enough calories to support that growth can lead to problems down the line.

Children, especially, should avoid weight cutting. They do not not have the ability to regulate body temperature to the same degree as adults through sweating. Cutting weight can also be psychologically detrimental and lead to eating disorders.

14. WEIGHT FLUCTUATIONS

Mostly all weight fluctuations are due to increased body-water content. Your body weight will fluctuate 1–2% daily due to differing levels of water content. You tend to weigh less first thing in the morning and more by the end of the day.

Daily weight gain can be caused by an increased intake of: water, fiber, sodium, or carbohydrates. It can also come from other factors, including: meal timing, hormones, edema, weather, elevation, or medications.

Daily weight loss can be caused by a decreased intake of water, fiber, sodium, or carbohydrates. It can also happen because of other factors, including: dehydration, illness, or gastrointestinal viruses. Daily weigh-ins can be utilized to better understand your body's weight fluctuations.

15. FINAL DEHYDRATION

How much weight you can lose during the final dehydration session before weigh-in depends on your size, age, sex, and other individual factors. Generally, losing more than 3–5% of your overall weight is not recommended during the final dehydration session.

16. BEING LEAN

Leaner individuals are able to cut more water out of the body. Humans beings are composed primarily of water; the average human body is approximately 60% water. This percentage is higher in athletes. Athletes tend to have less fat mass and more lean muscle. Fat contains about 10% water, while muscle contains about 70–80% water. Getting relatively lean allows for more water to be cut, leading to a greater competitive advantage.

17. WATER

Water in the body is distributed in predominantly three compartments: 1) Intracellularly, within the cell. 2) Extracellularly, outside of the cell. 3) As fluid in the blood.

Water also regulates body temperature through sweating. Water transports nutrients to the body and helps filter waste products from the body as it passes through the kidneys and is excreted as urine. Water aids digestion and lubricates joints.

18. DRY MOUTH

When you have dry mouth, there are several things you can do to increase saliva production; chewing dry-mouth gum, sucking on hard candies, using dry-mouth spray or mouth wash, or sucking on ice and then spitting out the water. Some athletes are able to tolerate dry mouth more than others, so find what works for you through experimentation.

19. RUNNING

Any old-school boxing trainer will tell you that one of the fundamentals is running—both for conditioning the body and mind, and for making weight.

Especially if you are relying primarily on active dehydration to make weight, running is essential. There is something about the human body that responds to running. I notice it right away in camp when an athlete has not put adequate time into their roadwork. Running improves athleticism, and high-level cardiovascular endurance is a must. Your cardio allows you to push the pace while keeping your technique sharp, but it also allows you to recover between rounds, between using bursts of energy, and from taking damage. Running is also one of the most effective ways to initiate active sweating.

A well-conditioned athlete can lose 3–5+ pounds in 30 to 40 minutes of running. There are plenty of athletes who do not use passive-dehydration methods for making weight, and running is one of the most tried-and-true methods.

20. JETLAG

You tend to experience jet lag when traveling across time zones. Generally, you need 24 hours to acclimate per time zone traveled. Caffeine and melatonin can be effective supplements for jet lag. Typically, 100–200 mg of caffeine can be used to stay awake when needed, and 0.3 to 1 mg of melatonin can be used prior to bedtime.

21. ALTITUDE

You typically need 14 to 21 days or longer to fully acclimate to elevation above 4000 ft. If you're unable to arrive that far in advance, aim for at least 5 to 7 days.

22. MENTAL

Everything begins and ends with desire. All things in your life are driven by your desire to be what you truly want to be. If you genuinely have the desire to be great, you will do what it takes. This doesn't mean that you will simply push harder and outwork everyone else. This doesn't mean that you will force outcomes to go your way. It means that you will do what is necessary to be effective in every situation that helps you get to your destination. Whether that's working harder than everyone else when it's needed, or taking a rest day when it's necessary. Greatness comes from your sincere desire to be great. Naturally, with desire comes the fear that you will not reach your destination. It is what it is.

Know that, when you are genuine in your pursuit, you tend to find your way. Things may even begin to happen that cannot be explained, which aid you in that process. Of course, there will be bumps in the road, and people may fall off along the way. But those who have a sufficient level of desire always tend to reach their destination.

ABOUT THE AUTHOR

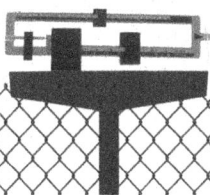

Coach **Ben Zee** is a performance coach to athletes in the UFC, Bellator, PFL, ONE, NHL, Professional Grappling, and Boxing.

Please visit coachbz.com